How To Choose
The Best Diet

LINDA LAZARIDES

Other works by Linda Lazarides

Principles of Nutritional Therapy
The Nutritional Health Bible
The Waterfall Diet
The Easy Water Retention Diet
Linda's Soup Diet Secrets
Linda's Flat Stomach Secrets
The Amino Acid Report
A Textbook of Modern Naturopathy

About the Author

Linda Lazarides is one of Britain's most respected natural health experts, and author of eight titles on health and nutrition. In 1996 she helped the University of Westminster to set up the UK's first degree course in Nutritional Therapy. She is founder of the British Association for Nutritional Therapy, former nutrition editor of the International Journal of Alternative & Complementary Medicine, Founder and Principal of the School of Modern Naturopathy, and for several years worked as a complementary practitioner for the British National Health Service.

Published by
The School of Modern Naturopathy
BCM Waterfall, London WC1N 3XX
www.modern-naturopathy.com

ISBN: 1716057717
ISBN-13: 978-1-716-05771-7

Printed and distributed by Lulu.com

DEDICATION

This book is dedicated to Professor John Yudkin, author of *Pure, White and Deadly*, who tried so many years ago to tell us about the dangers of excess sugar in our diet.

CONTENTS

FOREWORD

I wrote this book because I saw many social media arguments about whose diet was best. Whole-food plant-based dieters battled it out against those who claimed to feel wonderfully well eating little more than meat and butter. To be honest, I was shocked that diet books were out there recommending this.

Some people were so anxious to adhere to these books that they worried about consuming any carbohydrate calories at all, counting beans, lentils, carrots, apples and oats among foods to be avoided at all costs.

Others obsessed about fat avoidance, always dry-baking their food in air fryers without even one drop of olive oil.

This led me to debates about ketosis, revealing books by popular authors (some of them cardiologists and diabetes experts) to whom fans had given near-biblical status.

So who is right? Who should win the online arguments?

The only way to find out is to go to the medical databases and study the research. All of it. So that's what I did. This book is the result. I hope you will find it useful.

I would like to thank my readers for their invaluable feedback and support.

Linda Lazarides

1.
DO YOU HAVE
A DIET GURU?

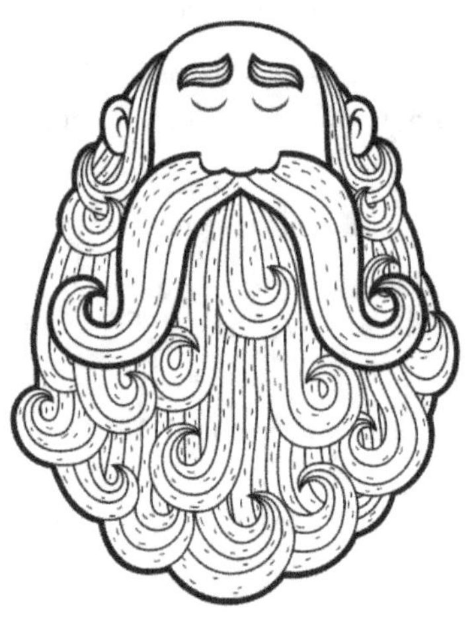

Diet fashions come and go, driven by the latest diet guru! In the 1970s the F-Plan Diet was all the rage. I followed it myself, and loved it. It was all about filling up on dietary fibre to eat less calories yet still feel satisfied. I added bran to every meal. My husband got pretty annoyed with me, especially when he had to ask to go to the toilet in the middle of a very important college exam!

It's a lot of fun trying out a new diet book. Everything makes so much sense, and if we do manage to lose some weight, we can get very attached to the diet; the author takes on a guru- like status, and people have been known to come to (verbal) blows in social media (lol). But, as always, beware. Things might not be as simple as the book would make it appear. The book may seem to be impeccably science-based, and quote lots of research studies; but every real scientist knows that for every research study that supports a dieting method, there is another that doesn't.

Sometimes that's because the various researchers are not comparing like with like. For instance, a "low-carb" diet (a diet where the carb intake is 50 grams per day or less) can cover an infinite number of food choices and combinations, some of them with a lot of fat or meat, others with very little. Some consisting only of whole-foods, others allowing sugar and refined flour.

Dieters in research studies may be incorporating factors from other dieting methods unknown to the researchers, such as skipping breakfast, avoiding gluten, or taking dietary supplements. Some will exercise more than others. Some will eat the same number of low calories every day, while others will have "binge" days that boost their metabolism.

So beware. An author wants to sell you a single "new" idea and will pick the research studies that fit that idea. Some of those studies may not even have used humans! Test animals like rats and mice are not equivalent to humans, and are simply not meant to be applied to us. If there are no human studies to back up the author's claims, it means that scientists didn't think the idea would work on humans.

2.
AGE MATTERS!

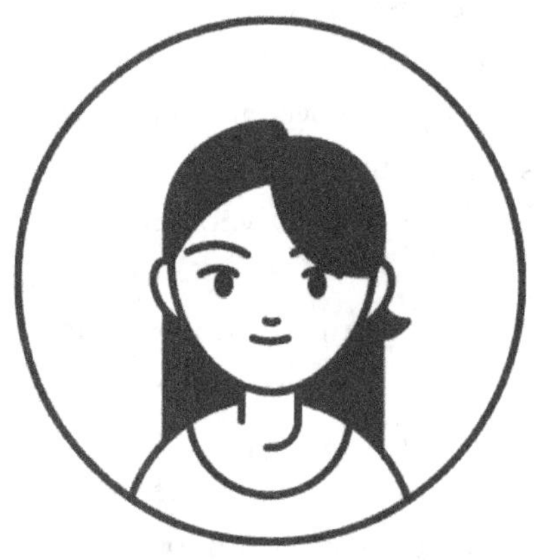

It is easy to lose weight up to middle age. It's a simple matter of calories-in, vs. calories-out. But once you hit your mid-40s, you will often find that doesn't work any more. Even a diet of only 1,000 Calories per day can leave you struggling with your weight. We usually put it down to a sedentary lifestyle and "middle-age spread".

The age factor is very poorly understood. Doctors and dieticians who put you on a low-calorie diet to lose weight frequently don't believe you are sticking to it if the diet doesn't work. Of course there are individuals who cheat, but I have had clients who were in despair because they ate so little and no-one would believe them.

3.
WATER RETENTION

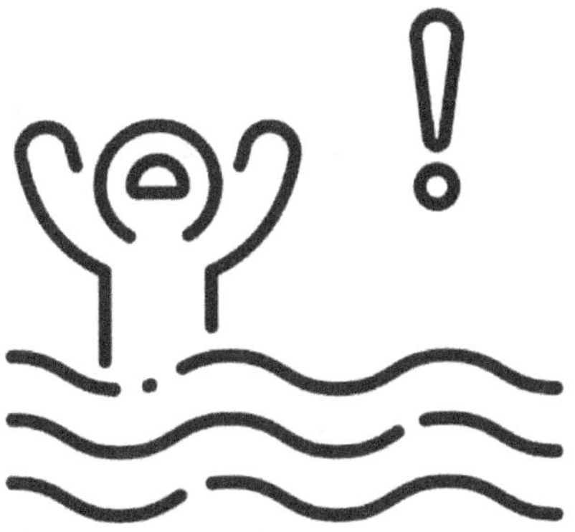

Not all excess weight is body fat. Hidden water retention looks like fat but cannot be shifted by eating fewer calories.

An intolerance (similar to an allergy) to a food like gluten, can cause inflammation that makes our tissues water-logged and heavy. If you start to avoid that food, you can pee out pounds of water weight. But as soon as you eat a little of it, water weight returns within days.

Several pounds of weight loss within a few days on a low-carb diet, probably has nothing to do with the carbs, and everything to do with avoiding gluten. By avoiding carbs you are also accidentally avoiding gluten.

4.
METABOLISM

You know you have a problem with metabolism when you only have to look at food to put on weight. Your metabolism is controlled by your thyroid gland. In turn, this gland is dependent on a number of vitamins and minerals that can be very short in the average diet. These include: Vitamins A and D Iron Zinc Iodine Selenium Vitamin A deficiency can be a vicious cycle. If your thyroid gland is underactive, you can't turn beta carotene from vegetables into proper vitamin A - also known as retinol. A retinol deficiency impairs the ability of the thyroid gland to do its work. Most people believe that taking iodine supplements will "boost" their thyroid gland and their metabolism. Although iodine deficiency is common, iodine supplements should not be taken without selenium. That's because most thyroid insufficiency is not caused by a lack of iodine but by an auto-immune condition known as autoimmune thyroiditis. Iodine supplements can make this condition worse unless you also take selenium to balance them. You can read more about this here: https://pubmed.ncbi.nlm.nih.gov/32588591/

Boosting your metabolism

One of the best ways to boost metabolism is to build muscle. The more muscle tissue you have, the more mitochondria. These are the energy-producing parts of your cells; the more mitochondria you have, the faster you will burn your calories. Muscles create mitochondria in response to demands on them, so the more you use your muscles, the better you will burn your calories. The best form of exercise is known as "interval training". This involves many short, strenuous bursts of exercise, with rests in between. During these rests your body will produce growth hormone, which rapidly burns fat!

Eating boosts metabolism!

One of the most important rules of dieting is not to diet every day. Your body quickly adapts to low-calorie eating, and adjusts its metabolism to burn calories more slowly. That's because it sees your fat stores as precious. It doesn't like to use them for energy. That's a survival mechanism against the threat of starvation. The result will be a weight "plateau". On a long-term low-calorie diet, weight loss will keep slowing down and then stop.

Weight loss plateau

Eating boosts the metabolism. If you break your low-calorie diet with a day of normal (let's call them "binge") meals, your metabolism will be higher and will burn calories and body fat much faster for about 24 hours before it starts to decline again over a four-day period. So you can avoid the dreaded plateau by eating normally once every four days, or maybe just one day a week. That means you can have a nice restaurant meal to look forward to at the weekend. If you fast and exercise vigorously the day after your binge, that temporary faster metabolism will ensure maximum fat burning.

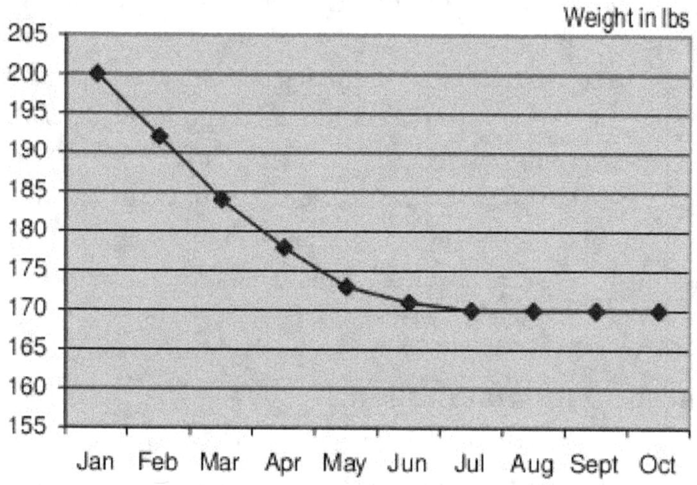

Weight Loss Plateau

5.
INTERMITTENT FASTING

The binge day technique is similar in some ways to a practice known as "intermittent fasting".

If you avoid food completely for about 12 hours, your body's carbohydrate stores will be exhausted and it will be forced to burn fat. In other words, it goes into a state of "ketosis", which means obtaining its energy from ketone bodies instead of from glucose and glycogen (forms of stored carbohydrate).

You can't burn fat if you eat soon after that 12 hours is up, because your body will use the food as an energy source instead, even if that meal doesn't contain any carbs. Glucose can be created from both fat and protein by your liver, in a process known as gluconeogenesis.

So if you want to burn body fat, you have to go without food for longer than 12 hours. Many popular books offer different plans for how to fit this into your life. I like the 16:8 plan - fasting for 16 hours, followed by eating all your meals within the remaining 8-hour window. So if your last food for the day is eaten at 7 pm, you can resume eating at 11 am the next day. Provided your "calories in" are equal to or less than your "calories out" for that day, you won't gain any more body fat. You will have a net loss of the amount of body fat you were able to burn between 7 am and 11 am. Cool! That would be a good time to exercise! But make sure you don't eat low-calorie every day. You still need a normal calorie intake day once a week to prevent the decline of your metabolic rate.

Another popular intermittent fasting plan is the 5:2 plan: eat normally 5 days a week. On the other 2 days (eg. Monday and Thursday) eat just one meal of about 500 calories. I recommend exercising on those days. Remember, you burn calories faster for 24 hours after a "binge" day.

Don't go too long without eating. Your body can become used to it and you will hit the dreaded plateau.

Ketone bodies are water-soluble molecules that contain the ketone groups produced from fatty acids by the liver. They are readily transported into tissues outside the liver, where they are converted into acetyl-CoA —which then enters the citric acid cycle and is oxidized for energy. Wikipedia

6.

IS FASTING GOOD FOR YOU?

Fasting won't just help you burn body fat, it stimulates an important process in the body known as autophagy. Literally meaning "self-eating", autophagy is the body's way of detoxing its own cells. When the food supply is short, our cells activate mechanisms to digest their own bad parts. It's a bit like when we didn't have time to go to the supermarket. Instead, we go to the fridge, looking for stuff to eat that's been hanging around a while and is past its sell-by date. For your cells, that's a great spring-clean which doesn't get done when food is in plentiful supply. It's the reason why the early naturopaths used to use fasting as a cancer treatment. They didn't know about the word "autophagy", but they believed that fasting could help the body eliminate its diseased parts. We don't know exactly how long you need to fast before autophagy starts. It is likely to be around 24 hours after food was last consumed, and it peaks after 48 hours of fasting.

You can also stimulate autophagy by eating a low-protein diet - especially a plant-based diet. By avoiding certain amino acids found mostly in animal products, you can fool the body into thinking it is fasting. Autophagy may be one of the reasons why a whole-food plant-based diet has such a positive healing effect when used against common diseases of old age. There is an amazing amount of research where a vegan diet has reversed problems such as high blood pressure, angina, congestive heart failure, kidney disease and osteoarthritis amongst others.

7.

SLOW METABOLISM AND WATER RETENTION

Below is an extract from my book *The Easy Water Retention Diet.*

Water retention increases the distance between blood vessels and cells in your body, and expands the tissue space between cells. It dilutes nutrients and oxygen, and damages cell-to-cell communication. Cell membranes become more permeable to toxins which they would not normally absorb.

One of the effects of this waterlogging is to slow down your metabolism, making it much harder for you to burn off your calories. People with water retention find that normal weight loss diets just don't work, or else they work up to a point, but the last 20 pounds or so just will not shift. Before you can boost your metabolism, you need to get rid of the water retention.

Here is another story from my casebook: Georgie, age 49, worked in a care home for people with Alzheimer's disease. She was eating as little as she could, and got plenty of exercise, being on her feet most days from 7 am until sometimes 9 pm, up and down stairs. But no matter how hard she tried, her weight would not budge from 12 stone (168 lbs). Worst of all, it was creeping slowly upwards although for the last four years she was eating little but salad with a small portion of lean grilled meat or fish, and thin wheat crackers. I wondered if Georgie suffered from hidden water retention, so I asked if any parts of her body felt swollen. She had not noticed any swellings, except for her knees. Georgie's doctor had diagnosed her with osteoarthritis because her knees were painful and swollen, made much worse by walking upstairs. Marjorie had to take painkillers every day for her knee pains.

There was such a lot of swelling around both Georgie's knees that it didn't really make sense unless it was related to a more general body water retention problem. I told Georgie that I believed she suffered from hidden water retention in other parts of her body, and that there was only one way to find out - to try my water retention diet (also known as the Waterfall Diet) on an experimental basis. Georgie was keen to try anything if it could help her lose weight, and started the diet immediately. After a few days, I got an excited phone call. 'I think I've been suffering from water retention all these years' she said. 'I've been peeing it all away - several gallons so far. My clothes are so loose they're hanging off me!'

Georgie peed so much that she weighed 15 lbs less by the end of the first week on my diet. The peeing and weight loss stopped for a few days, and then started again. Two weeks later when she saw me again, she was ecstatic. 'I've been constantly on the loo again and have lost another 7 lbs. My knee swelling has disappeared, the pains have completely gone, I no longer need painkillers, and I'm feeling so full of energy for the first time in years that I'm going to start an exercise class!

Georgie lost a total of 22 lbs of water retention, and as long as she didn't eat the wrong foods, it never came back again. Within a few short months she was looking 10 years younger. After getting rid of the excess water, Georgie's metabolism had improved so much that she also managed to lose a few pounds of body fat, something that was not possible while her body was waterlogged. Georgie was my most successful case ever.

Sadly, so many doctors won't believe people when they say they have been working hard at dieting. Some will more or less accuse you of stuffing yourself with chocolate bars and just not admitting it. I have known people driven to the verge of tears because they were already on a starvation diet, but instead of getting slimmer they were getting fatter.

Don't be one of these people. The diet in this book may be the answer for you, so don't lose hope.

From The Easy Water Retention Diet, by Linda Lazarides.

Do not be tempted to take diuretic meds like Lasix for water retention unless your doctor has prescribed them for a heart or kidney condition. If your doctor doesn't know what's causing your water retention then you have what is known as the "idiopathic" type. Diuretics usually make this type worse. My book The *Easy Water Retention Diet* explains why.

8.
OVER-EATING

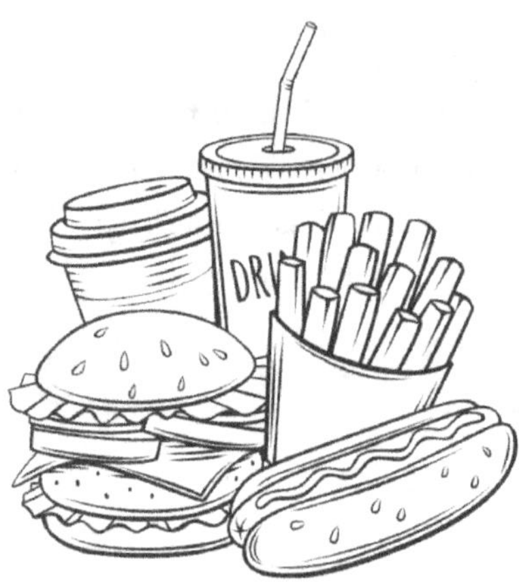

Before you decide on a diet, it's important to think about how you became overweight in the first place.

Do you use food to relieve boredom or stress? Or do you have a food addiction, such as chocolate or pizza? You may need to change your life before you can let go of the cookie jar. A change of job, partner, a new interest, going back to school, or even moving to a new country, can all help to fill that spiritual black hole that food will never be able to fill.

If the cause of your over-eating isn't addressed, it's very likely you will just be a "yo-yo" dieter; eating salads for a week, then giving in to temptation and putting the weight straight back on again.

The most difficult thing with weight control is to keep the weight off after you have lost it. If you go back to your previous dietary habits, you will go back to your previous weight, and perhaps even a little more. As I've already said, prolonged low-calorie eating slows down the metabolism.

Some people over-eat because they feel hungry all the time, even if they have only just eaten. This is likely due to "leptin resistance". Leptin is the satiety hormone. Internal abdominal fat (the kind that grows around your organs and gives your stomach an apple or beer gut shape) produces a leptin neutralizer which stops your body from detecting leptin. This is why morbidly obese people are often permanently hungry.

In theory you should be able to reduce your production of leptin neutralizer (its proper name is C-reactive protein) by losing excess internal abdominal fat. So as you burn off body fat, it is to be hoped that your appetite will return to normal. Vitamin C supplements may also be able to reduce C-reactive protein, but scientists don't know whether these supplements can also help prevent you feeling hungry all the time.

Occasionally, children can be born without the ability to make leptin, and they start to become morbidly obese from a very early age.

9.
SOUP DIETING

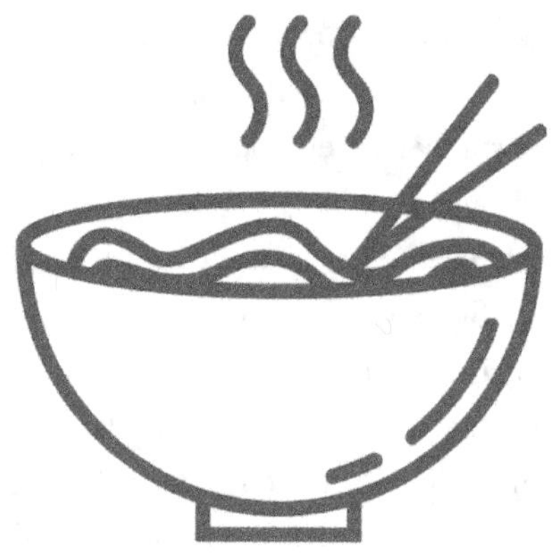

Soup dieting was made popular by books about the "Cabbage Soup Diet" that originated in China. I made a study of the cabbage soup diet, and discovered that the soup in question is really a vegetable hodge-podge, and that cabbage itself doesn't have any magic weight-loss properties! But soup dieting is an extremely effective technique for over-eaters and people with a large appetite. It's actually quite a simple principle, and there are several research studies which explain how it works.

Basically, the addition of warm liquid to food bulks out the meal so you feel satisfied on less calories. It also slows down the digestion of that meal, causing it to stay in the digestive system for longer. As a result, the people in the research studies felt full for much longer, and ate less at the next meal.

If your soup happens to be a hodge-podge of vegetables, especially cabbage, it will also be loaded with dietary fibre that, like water, bulks out your meal with even more zero calories. So the end effect of the cabbage soup diet is that your meals will be satisfying despite being quite low in calories. You will also not feel the need to eat as much quantity. If you get hungry, you can happily go back for more helpings of soup, knowing that the calorie content is minimal.

Soup is also very easy to make, so it's perfect for people who don't do much home cooking. You can make a large batch to last for several days and just heat it up. I myself eat a lot of home-made mixed vegetable soups to help control my weight, and I find they really help. If you're interested in learning more about soup dieting, I wrote a whole book about it, with recipes. The title is *Linda's Soup Diet Secrets*.

9.
CARBOHYDRATES

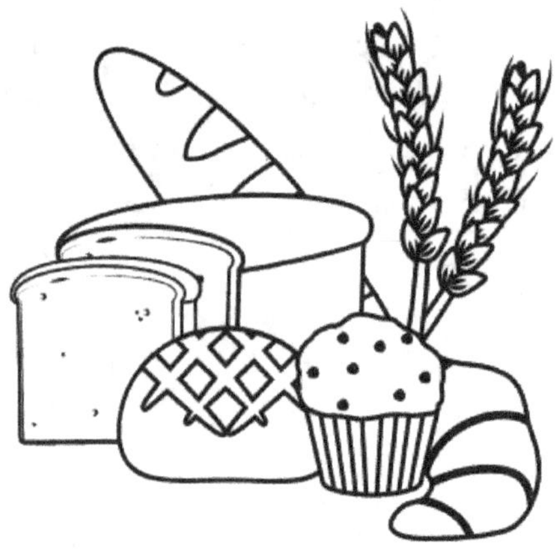

All over the world people use big portions of starchy food: rice, pasta, bread or potatoes to "fill up". Athletes are recommended to get the bulk of their energy from these so-called "complex carbs". Perhaps the only cultures that developed without this tradition were the Eskimos, with their diets of fish, meat and blubber, and the ancient hunter-gatherer tribes like those in the Amazon rainforest, who traditionally live on small animals, fruit and tree-foods.

Eating meat and starch is considered to be part of the natural diet of humans, one we have adapted to over thousands of years. But evolution is measured in millions of years, not thousands. Three million years ago, humans did not have tools. They did not grow crops, and they could not hunt large animals. Their diet would have been restricted very much to what primates still eat today. Primates are our closest relatives in the animal kingdom. Perhaps we should be eating a "Primate Diet" of fruit, flowers, leaves, nuts, bark, pith, seeds, grasses, roots, birds' eggs, small rodents, frogs and insects? Perhaps that is really what we are designed for? If this was our diet, we would have to eat much larger quantities of food to get our needed calories. Primates in the wild spend a large part of their day foraging for food. With those greater quantities of whole, natural foods, think how much higher, calorie-for-calorie, would be our intake of vitamins, minerals and phytonutrients, compared with a bowl of rice?

Based on the researches I have been doing in regard to the human ageing process, I have a theory that we have to pay a price for every calorie we consume in the form of sugar, refined starch or fat. I would personally add large-animal meat to that list, for reasons you will find out in the scientific research summaries provided later on. I say "large animal" because our ancestors would have consumed a whole mouse or frog, providing far more nutrients than beef or chicken muscle meat, for instance.

The price I'm referring to is something that in the science of ageing, is called "cell senescence". It is responsible for all our diseases of old age. Our modern diet may appear to keep us healthy, but only while we are young, My online video course on cell senescence can be found at www.udemy.com/course/body-rejuvenation-therapy/

10.
CARBOHYDRATES AND INSULIN

Carbohydrates in the form of starch and sugar stimulate our body's production of the hormone insulin. We need insulin to extract glucose from our blood into our cells, where it can be converted to energy. (NB: All carbs are broken down by the digestive process into simple sugars like glucose.)

But persistently high insulin due to a diet that is constantly high in sugar and starch but short on many essential vitamins and minerals, can lead to a condition known as insulin resistance. In insulin resistance, the body becomes less sensitive to insulin, so insulin doesn't remove enough glucose from the blood. The body may then produce more insulin in an attempt to overcome this, resulting in chronically high insulin levels.

But some organs cannot cope with this extra insulin. Too much insulin makes the kidneys retain sodium, causing water retention, high blood pressure and high levels of uric acid. When insulin over-stimulates the liver, blood fats (triglycerides) rise, leading to heart and artery disease. A woman's ovaries can begin making more testosterone, leading to symptoms of polycystic ovary syndrome (PCOS).

Another effect of high insulin is a change in body shape. As we head into middle age, body fat begins to collect mainly inside the abdomen increasing our weight and our girth at the front of the waist. It is very, very hard to lose.

High insulin levels also encourage the formation of inflammatory prostaglandins, which can promote the development of degenerative diseases.

These facts are the foundation for the recent trend towards "low-carb diets". They aim to control our production of insulin and so make it easier to lose weight.

11.
LOW-CARB DIETS

A whole industry has grown up around the concept of low-carb dieting. The general rule is: control your insulin by eating protein and fat instead of carbs. If you make less insulin, you'll lose weight more easily. As a rule, they say, no more than 50 grams of carbs per day are permitted, but some authors don't even allow that!

Hopefully your favourite low-carb author knows that controlling insulin isn't all about carb avoidance. Naturopaths warn that we must also get an adequate intake of B vitamins and the trace element chromium, that are essential for insulin sensitivity. The better our insulin sensitivity, the less insulin we need to make. It is even possible that people develop insulin resistance partly because they have a long-term deficiency of those nutrients. They are mostly found in whole-foods like oats, nuts and legumes.

So your diet guru wants you to eat protein and fat instead of carbs? Are you seeing bottles of oil, hunks of meat and packs of butter and cheese? A low-carb diet consists of steak, fish, cheese, chicken and butter, right?

Well, it actually depends on which author or guru you believe. Some want you to be a carnivore and eat nothing except animal products. Others say you can add some vegetables to your meat and fat, like leafy greens.

It all seems good sense, and no doubt the author is highly qualified and provides lots of stories and research proving weight loss success. But a little knowledge can be a dangerous thing, and later on I'll be showing you some studies that maybe your favourite diet author didn't know about, or simply didn't tell you...

After all, you don't want to swap one health problem for another!

12.
KETOGENIC DIETS

Also known as "keto" diets, these are based on the principle that if you avoid eating carbs, and replace them with fat, you will start to burn your body fat. In order to do this, your liver has to convert fatty acids into "ketone bodies" which can be transported into other tissues and converted into acetyl-CoA. Acetyl-CoA is a molecule which is able to enter the same energy production pathway as glucose, to make energy. When your body is undergoing this process, it is said to be in a state of "ketosis". Ketogenic diets have been around a very long time, and were first used as a natural treatment for epilepsy.

As for what you eat, keto diets are similar to low-carb diets. You are not allowed more than 30 to 50 grams of carbs per day, and all the rest of your calories must come from fat and protein, particularly fat (70-80 per cent).

The official Recommended Daily Amount of protein (about 50 grams per day) should not be exceeded, since too much protein can interfere with ketosis.

Unlike fasting, where ketosis is said to start at around 12 hours, a keto diet requires several days for the body to enter into the ketosis state.

For maximum weight loss a keto diet should also be low in calories. In medical research, this combination is known as a VLCKD (very low-calorie ketogenic diet). I will provide summaries of research reviews about the long-term safety of these diets. The fact that people with epilepsy are prescribed a non-VLC keto diet to control their disease is not the same as self-administering a VLCKD diet for weight control on a long-term basis. We need a wide variety of plant antioxidants and phytonutrients to help to protect us from age- related diseases.

13.
YOUR MICROBIOTA

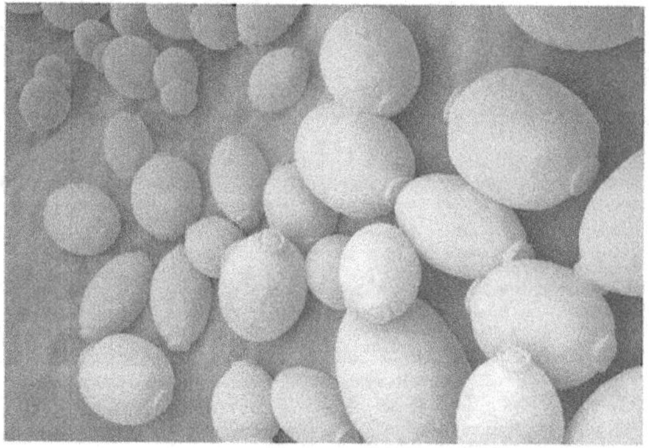

If you're feeling incredibly well on your low-carb/ketogenic or carnivore diet, there can be a reason that naturopaths are well aware of but few others are. Your microbiota may have been out of balance.

The microbiota is the population of resident bacteria and yeasts that live permanently in your gut. Some of these micro-organisms, like Acidophilus and Bifidobacteria, are friendly and beneficial. Others can become very toxic if the friendly ones fail to keep them under control.

The Candida yeast pictured on the previous page is one of these. If it gets out of control, It can form a highly toxic fungal overgrowth in our intestines.Candida albicans

The initial symptoms of Candida intestinal overgrowth are bloating and gas, eventually leading to a persistent hangover-like, "tired-all-the-time" feeling, and increasing food intolerances, inflammation such as skin rashes, and nutritional deficiencies as the yeast overgrowth hinders nutrient absorption.

Candida albicans is found everywhere. When in small enough numbers to be controlled by the friendly gut micro-organisms, it does no harm. But the population of these friendly bacteria is decimated whenever you take antibiotics. Yeasts, on the other hand, are not affected by antibiotics.

Just like the yeasts used in breweries, Candida lives off sugar - in this case the sugar that awaits digestion in your intestines. Starch (eg. white flour) is turned into sugar too. Candida uses sugar to make alcohol and the toxic by-product acetaldehyde. So your diet can encourage Candida to make you feel very ill indeed.

If you eliminate sugar and starch from your diet, the yeast will have trouble surviving, and will start to die off. So will your bloating, fatigue, headaches and inflammatory symptoms. So amongst other things, naturopaths prescribe a low-carb diet to control Candida.

The microbiota can also be unbalanced by a high-meat diet and the lack of a wide variety of plant foods. Research shows that the microbiota associated with this kind of diet is linked with a higher rate of age-related diseases.

There are more bacteria in our intestines than there are cells in our body. They are producing a variety of substances, both toxic and non-toxic, all the time, which are absorbed into our blood and travel around our body. So getting the right balance of microbiota is very important.

14.
WHAT THE RESEARCHERS SAY

I looked up all the most recent weight loss diet papers in the medical databases covering research on humans, and found these results.

1. Eliminating starch and sugar works better than eliminating fat Temple, N.J. Fat, Sugar, Whole Grains and Heart Disease: 50 Years of Confusion. Nutrients 2018, 10, 39.

During the 1970s only a few scientists, including British Professor John Yudkin, author of *Pure, White and Deadly*, believed that refined carbohydrates (especially sugar) and a low intake of dietary fibre, were major factors in coronary heart disease (CHD). The official view, which lasted from roughly 1974 to 2014, was that an excess intake of saturated fat was the key factor. But findings since 1990 inform us that the role of saturated fat in the development of CHD has been much exaggerated. The evidence linking carbohydrate-rich foods and especially sugar-sweetened beverages, with CHD, has been steadily strengthening. On the other hand, whole grains and cereal fiber are protective. An extra 1-2 servings per day of these foods decreases risk by approximately 10 to 20 per cent.

www.mdpi.com/2072-6643/10/1/39/htm

2. Research that obtained positive results using a keto diet for obesity, in people with or without type 2 diabetes

Bueno N, et al, 2013. Very-low-carbohydrate ketogenic diet v. low-fat diet for long-term weight loss: A meta-analysis of randomised controlled trials. British Journal of Nutrition, 110(7), 1178-1187.

https://pubmed.ncbi.nlm.nih.gov/23651522/

Bhanpuri, N.H., et al. Cardiovascular disease risk factor responses to a type 2 diabetes care model including nutritional ketosis induced by sustained carbohydrate restriction at 1 year: an open label, non-randomized, controlled study. Cardiovasc Diabetol 17, 56 (2018).

https://cardiab.biomedcentral.com/articles/10.1186/s12933-018-0698-8

Goday A, Bellido D, Sajoux I, et al. Short-term safety, tolerability and efficacy of a very-low-calorie ketogenic diet interventional weight loss program versus hypocaloric diet in patients with type 2 diabetes mellitus. Nutr Diabetes. 2016;6(9):e230. Published 2016 Sep 19.

www.ncbi.nlm.nih.gov/pmc/articles/PMC5048014/ Gomez-Arbelaez D, et al Body Composition Changes After Very-Low-Calorie Ketogenic Diet in Obesity Evaluated by 3 Standardized Methods. J Clin Endocrinol Metab. 2017 Feb 1;102(2):488-498.

https://pubmed.ncbi.nlm.nih.gov/27754807/

It is understandable why reading about this research may get you excited if you are keen to lose weight and have already tried other diets. But below is a meta-analysis - a study which compares the results found in ALL the studies and trials carried out to date on this topic. Meta-analyses are very important because scientists know that for every trial which shows a positive result, there will be another that doesn't! Only by weighing up both sides do we have a chance of arriving at the truth.

3. A meta-analysis of ketogenic diets: safety and efficacy Crosby L, Davis B, Joshi S, et al. Ketogenic Diets and Chronic Disease: Weighing the Benefits Against the Risks. Front Nutr. 2021;8:702802. Published 2021 Jul 16.

Ketogenic diets reduce seizure frequency in some individuals with epilepsy. These diets can also reduce body weight, although not more effectively than other dietary approaches over the long term or when matched for calorie intake. Ketogenic diets can also lower blood glucose, although their efficacy typically wanes after a few months. Very-low-carbohydrate diets are associated with marked risks. LDL-C cholesterol can rise, sometimes dramatically. Pregnant women on such diets are more likely to have a child with a neural tube type birth defect, even when supplementing folic acid. These diets may increase chronic disease risk: foods and dietary components that typically increase on ketogenic diets (eg. red meat, processed meat, saturated fat) are linked to an increased risk of kidney disease, cardiovascular disease, cancer, diabetes, and Alzheimer's disease, whereas the intake of protective foods (eg. vegetables, fruits, legumes, whole grains) typically decreases. Current evidence suggests that for most individuals, the risks of such diets outweigh the benefits.
www.ncbi.nlm.nih.gov/pmc/articles/PMC8322232/

One of the risks is ketoacidosis, which can be life-threatening. A keto diet properly designed need not raise your acidity levels more than a normal diet does, but some individuals get a little "weight-loss greedy" and are not aware of the risks. Here's a case reported in a medical journal.

Blanco JC, et al. Starvation Ketoacidosis due to the Ketogenic Diet and Prolonged Fasting - A Possibly Dangerous Diet Trend. Am J Case Rep. 2019;20:1728-1731. Published 2019 Nov 22.

A ketogenic diet can be modified by the addition of intermittent or prolonged fasting which will also restrict calorie intake. In certain conditions, this ketosis can develop into overt ketoacidosis, leading to serious illness and hospitalization. Besides ketoacidosis, a ketogenic diet may lead to electrolyte abnormalities, hypoglycemia, acute pancreatitis, and dyslipidemia. In this case, a 60-year-old male with a history of type 2 diabetes, was following a ketogenic diet and also engaging in intermittent fasting. After 5 days of fasting, the patient ate some soup and began to vomit and become dizzy. He collapsed and lost consciousness. Laboratory tests revealed ketoacidosis.

www.ncbi.nlm.nih.gov/pmc/articles/PMC6883983/

15.
ACID-ALKALINE BALANCE

The body's acid/alkaline balance is a profundly important health factor. It is measured in pH. Values of pH 0 to 6.9 indicate acidity, while values above 7 indicate alkalinity. The body works hard to keep our blood as close as possible to 7.4.

Urine pH is also significant. French scientist Professor Louis-Claude Vincent (1906-1988) discovered that urine pH seems to be lower in the presence of degenerative disease. Naturopaths reason that helping their clients work towards achieving a more ideal urine pH must be therapeutic.

High-protein foods can also raise levels of uric acid. On the other hand, fruits and vegetables, even if acidic in flavour, leave an alkaline residue so they help to neutralize excessive acid. Blueberries, cherries and celery are exceptionally helpful for reducing uric acid.

But food is not the only cause of excessive acidity in the body. Exposure to toxins and pollutants also contributes. Using enzymes, the liver's job is to transform undesirables in the blood into end-products which can be excreted by the kidneys. These end-products take the form of acids. Undesirables include not just obvious toxins, but also items such as medications, fumes and alcohol, and toxic waste products of intestinal bacteria, which are absorbed into the blood.

As acids build up, the blood is liable to stagnate. Just as milk curdles when a few drops of lemon juice are added to it, excessive acidity can increase the clotting tendency of blood and restrict the supply of oxygen. This is why you will often read in naturopathic texts that hyper-acidity causes oxygen starvation.

To prevent acidosis (acid poisoning) the body tries to raise pH by making the kidneys produce bicarbonate. Young, healthy kidneys can cope. But as we age, our kidneys become less efficient; acids that cannot be neutralized become deposited in the tissue spaces between the cells. Professor Vincent believed that the resulting "connective tissue acidosis' leads to the development of chronic degenerative diseases and cancers. Hyper-acidity is also likely to disturb the electrolyte balance, and thus the electrical activity of the heart and nervous system, and to promote osteoporosis - the thinning of the bones.

It is thought that connective tissue acidity can be estimated by measuring the pH of the urine after a 14-hour fast. Urine pH can be measured with dip sticks that are available cheaply from pharmacies or online. As you can see from the table on the previous page, a value of 6.8 is ideal. Anything below 6.0 is cause for concern.

Treatment of hyper-acidity

Since fruits and vegetables are metabolized to an alkaline residue, naturopaths often ask clients with degenerative conditions to avoid all other foods for two weeks. Fruits and vegetables and their juices also have the advantage of being high in potassium and magnesium, which can become depleted under conditions of excessive tissue acidity. This diet, perhaps with the addition of saunas to encourage elimination through the skin, aims to release acidic residues from connective tissue. Repeated testing of the urine pH can be used to monitor the results.

Plant protein foods such as nuts, beans, oats and tofu are low in acid-forming amino acids, and should be added to the diet after 1-2 weeks.

Gut pH

The small intestine and colon are a separate environment from the blood and tissues, and have their own needs. While an acidic urine is a bad sign, an acidic bowel pH helps to prevent colon cancer. It also helps to solubilize minerals, aiding their absorption from the colon. Beneficial gut bacteria such as Lactobacilli consume the dietary fibre from fruits and vegetables, producing short-chain fatty acids (SCFAs) which increase bowel acidity. SCFAs are also an important source of energy for the cells of the colon wall. In fact, dietary fibre is like a probiotic; friendly bacteria thrive by consuming it, and their numbers increase.

The British Journal of Cancer has reported that an alkaline colon pH increases the risk of colon cancer. It also encourages intestinal bacteria to turn hydrogen gas into "rotten egg gas". But under acidic colon conditions, hydrogen is instead turned to highly beneficial acetate by acetogenic bacteria. Gibson GR, Cummings JH et al. Alternative pathways for hydrogen disposal during fermentation in the human colon. Gut 1990 Jun;31(6):679-83.

Acetaldehyde

Acetaldehyde was mentioned in the section on the microbiota, and is considered to be one of the most potent triggers for colon cancer. Alcohol consumed in food or drink, or produced by fermentation in the colon, is converted to acetaldehyde by intestinal bacteria. These bacteria produce acetaldehyde much more vigorously when the pH of the colon is alkaline rather than neutral or acidic. Nosova T, Jousimies-Somer H. Characteristics of alcohol dehydrogenases of certain aerobic bacteria representing human colonic flora. Alcohol Clin Exp Res 1997 May;21 (3):489-94.

16.
WHOLE-FOOD PLANT-BASED DIETS

A whole-food plant-based (WFPB) diet consists of natural, unrefined plant foods such as whole-grains, nuts and beans, and excludes all animal products. It has low levels of acid-promoting amino acids. In the past, nutritionists used to believe that because of these low levels, plant proteins were "second-class" and animal products were "first-class" protein sources.

This concept dates back to the 1950s, and is very much out of date. Plants have a healthier balance of amino acids than meat, provided we eat a good variety of whole-foods. We really don't need a lot of protein to remain healthy. Although official figures advise an intake of about 50 grams of protein per day, some research suggests that we would be better off with no more than 20 to 30 grams. In a clinical study on 100 patients it was found that individuals who eat more than 30 grams per day of protein generate high levels of acid which must be neutralized by the kidneys before being eliminated. The authors concluded that a "normal" daily protein consumption is excessive, and conducive to ill health. Morter, M. Panfili, A. The Body's Negative Response to Excess Dietary Protein. J. Orthomolecular Med Vol. 13, 2nd Quarter 1998. http://orthomolecular.org/library/jom/1998/pdf/1998-v13n02-p089.pdf

The chart on the next page shows the protein content of some common plant foods.

I am astounded by the number of research studies in which people with age-related diseases have reversed them with a WFPB diet. You will find a list of these studies on my Modern Naturopathy website.

I can vouch for this myself. After a recent kidney test I discovered that my kidney function is poor. This was not good news; it means that my kidneys have been under excessive stress. I switched to a whole-food plant-based diet and my kidney function quickly rose by seven points.

Kidney function declines with age, and poor kidney function is the top cause of artery calcification and heart/artery disease (you can look this up - it's absolutely true but rarely mentioned by doctors). Everyone over the

age of 50 should get their kidney function tested every few years, and consider prolonging the healthy lifespan of their kidneys and heart by reducing their intake of animal protein.

The WFPB diet is essentially vegan, with the difference that many vegans rely heavily on commercial products that imitate items like meat and cheese. These imitation foods are not whole-foods; they can be very poor in nutritional value.

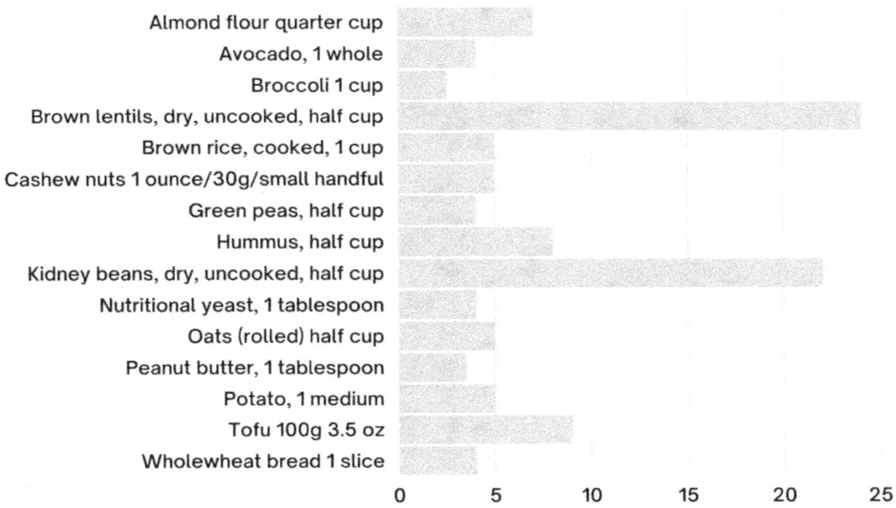

Protein Content of Plant Foods in grams

The adult daily protein requirement is 30 grams https://bit.ly/morter-panfili-protein-study

Peas, beans, lentils, nuts, tofu, nutritional yeast, whole-grains and potatoes all contain protein. To get enough protein it is not necessary to eat any animal products at all.

However we do recommend seeking out foods that have been fortified with vitamins B12 and D, or taking supplements, since plant-based foods are lacking in these nutrients.

Is a WFPB diet good for weight loss?

Researchers seem to think so. Here are summaries of some of the reviews and studies:

By "walling off your calories," preferentially deriving your macronutrients from structurally intact plant foods, some calories remain trapped within indigestible cell walls, which then blunts the glycemic impact and delivers prebiotics to the gut micro-biome. This may help explain why the current evidence indicates that a whole-food, plant-based diet achieves greater weight loss compared with other dietary interventions that do not restrict calories or mandate exercise. So, the most effective diet for weight loss appears to be the only diet shown to reverse heart disease in the majority of patients. Plant-based diets have also been found to help treat, arrest, and reverse other leading chronic diseases such as type 2 diabetes and hypertension, whereas low-carbohydrate diets have been found to impair artery function and worsen heart disease.

Greger M. A Whole Food Plant-Based Diet Is Effective for Weight Loss: The Evidence. Am J Lifestyle Med. 2020; 14(5):500-510. Published 2020 Apr 3.

www.ncbi.nlm.nih.gov/pmc/articles/PMC7444011/

A WFPB diet can also be made low-calorie and low-carb, and can be combined with intermittent fasting for even better results. Low-carb doesn't have to mean less than 50 grams of carbs per day or avoiding good foods like carrots and lentils because they contain a little carbohydrate. The important thing is to exclude refined starches and sugars.

Here is a study which compared what people ate, with their waist measurement. 847 subjects at high cardiovascular risk were recruited. Their consumption of meat or nuts was recorded and their waist measurements were taken. People with a lower body mass index and waist circumference were found to have a higher nut consumption. People with a larger waist circumference were found to have a higher meat consumption. Each 30g serving of nuts per day seems to reduce the BMI and waist circumference by 0.78 kg/m2 and 2.1 cm, respectively.

Casas-Agustench P, et al. Cross-sectional association of nut intake with adiposity in a Mediterranean population. Nutr Metab Cardiovasc Dis. 2011 Jul;21(7):518-25.

www.nmcd-journal.com/article/S0939-4753(09)00288-9/fulltext

Another study found that people with insulin resistance and central obesity tended to eat more red meat.

Babio N, et al. Association between red meat consumption and metabolic syndrome in a Mediterranean population at high cardiovascular risk: cross-sectional and 1-year follow-up assessment. Nutr Metab Cardiovasc Dis. 2012 Mar; 22(3):200-7.

www.nmcd-journal.com/article/S0939-4753(10)00165-1/fulltext

Remember autophagy, mentioned in the section on fasting? You can also trigger the autophagy process by only restricting protein consumption. Even just avoiding methionine - one of the main acid-promoting amino acids - will do the job. Methionine is found primarily in animal products.

17.
A FINAL WORD ABOUT MEAT

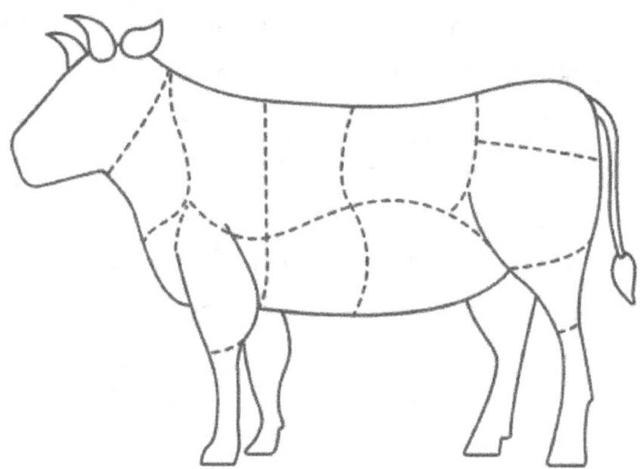

I know some of my readers will be sceptical about "anti-meat" research. The Carnivore Diet and its fore--runner the Paleo Diet are popular! Authors of carnivore dieting promise weight loss, improved mood, and blood sugar regulation. They tell convincing stories to back up these statements. But if you have been around a long while like I have, you will know how to see the holes in the arguments.

It's most likely to be just the avoidance of starch and sugar that makes you feel better and lose weight on these diets.

But a carnivore diet might also make you feel better if you:
- Suffer from a Candida albicans infestation
- Have an iron deficiency (meat is a good source of iron)
- Have an allergy or intolerance to gluten, dairy products, or eggs. Food intolerances can cause some pretty nasty symptoms like arthritis, migraine, eczema, irritable bowel syndrome, sometimes even asthma. Avoiding the offending food makes you feel amazing. If that's the case, don't credit meat with doing it for you! Most of us don't know that we have a food intolerance until we totally stop eating that food.

Hopefully you're beginning to doubt the health claims for a diet of meat and fat. It might not make you ill within the next year or two, but by the time you notice something is wrong, harmful changes may have already started. It is not for nothing that the World Health Organization has, since 1992 advised that eating more than two portions a week of red or processed meat increases the risk of colon cancer by as much as 20-30 per cent.
www.ncbi.nlm.nih.gov/pmc/articles/PMC4698595/

Compounds produced by the browning of meat and fat during the cooking process are thought to promote both cancer and diabetes. The acidity from a diet high in animal protein also causes minerals to leach out of bones. In later life this results in osteoporosis (brittle bones and shrinking of the spine).

18.
FATS

With so much emphasis in recent diet books about replacing carbohydrates with fats, it's time to take a closer look at the pros and cons of the different fats in our diet.

Fats have traditionally been looked at in broad categories: saturated, mono-unsaturated, and poly-unsaturated fat, but this is proving to be less and less relevant.

Fats consist of fatty acids attached to glycerol. When carb stores in the body run out, glycerol in fat can be converted to glucose.

Fatty acids are chains of carbon atoms with hydrogen atoms attached to them. In some fatty acids, pairs of carbon atoms are attached to each other by "double bonds" instead of to hydrogen atoms. These are known as unsaturated fatty acids. Depending on the number of double bonds, they are either mono-unsaturated (MUFA) or polyunsaturated (PUFA). The more double bonds, the more liquid the fat, Saturated fatty acids (SFA) are those without double bonds, and are solid at room temperature.

Nowadays research is trending towards looking at specific fatty acids. Here is a table showing the most common ones.

Saturated fatty acids	Unsaturated fatty acids
Lauric Acid	Linoleic acid* (n-6)
Myristic Acid	Alpha-linolenic acid* (n-3)
Palmitic Acid	Arachidonic acid
Stearic Acid	Oleic acid
*Classed as "essential" because they are needed for health but must be obtained from the diet (they cannot be made by the body). n=omega	

Scientists are also beginning to realize that the "matrix" - ie. whether the fatty acid is found in milk, meat or plant foods - also makes a difference. Here are some recent research studies:

Visioli F, Poli A. Fatty Acids and Cardio-vascular Risk. Evidence, Lack of Evidence, and Diligence. Nutrients. 2020;12(12):3782.
Fatty acids are part of more complex food matrices therefore, it is difficult to single out the contribution of individual classes of these compounds to human health. The same fatty acid ingested as part of a plant-based diet versus an animal-based often appears to exert different effects, even though it is difficult to explain such differences considering their obvious chemical identity.
www.ncbi.nlm.nih.gov/pmc/articles/PMC7764656/

Zong, Geng et al. Monounsaturated fats from plant and animal sources in relation to risk of coronary heart disease among US men and women. The American journal of clinical nutrition vol. 107,3 (2018): 445-453.
We investigated the associations of MUFA intake from plant and animal sources with coronary heart disease risk separately among 63,442 women from the Nurses' Health Study (1990–2012) and 29,942 men from the Health Professionals Follow-Up Study (1990–2012). The results we obtained suggest that plant foods are the preferable sources of MUFAs for coronary heart disease prevention.
www.ncbi.nlm.nih.gov/pmc/articles/PMC5875103/

19.
SATURATED FAT

I think everyone would agree that whatever weight control plan you use in the long term, you don't want it to accelerate the development of age-related diseases. Otherwise you are just swapping one problem for another. Scientists in the cardiology, diabetology and weight-loss fields recently seem to be quite keen to tell us it's ok to eat lots of saturated fat; that there's nothing wrong with it after all. But if these doctors had been a bit more diligent in their googling, they might not have been so quick to reach this conclusion (and to make a pile of money writing best-sellers).

Sure, there are some studies that show no harmful effects on the heart from eating saturated fat, but when researchers carried out a systematic review (a study comparing results from ALL the studies), this is what they found:

Clifton PM, Keogh JB. A systematic review of the effect of dietary saturated and polyunsaturated fat on heart disease. Nutr Metab Cardiovasc Dis. 2017 Dec;27(12):1060-1080.
Replacing saturated fat with PUFA, MUFA or high-quality carbohydrate will lower coronary heart disease events.
https://linkinghub.elsevier.com/retrieve/pii/S0939- 4753(17)30237-5

von Frankenberg AD, et al. A high-fat, high-saturated fat diet decreases insulin sensitivity without changing intra-abdominal fat in weight-stable overweight and obese adults. Eur J Nutr. 2017;56(1):431-443.
A diet very high in fat and saturated fat adversely affects insulin sensitivity and thereby might contribute to the development of type 2 diabetes.
www.ncbi.nlm.nih.gov/pmc/articles/PMC5291812/

DiNicolantonio JJ, O'Keefe JH. Good Fats versus Bad Fats: A Comparison of Fatty Acids in the Promotion of Insulin Resistance, Inflammation, and Obesity. Mo Med. 2017; 114(4):303-307.
Recently, debate has erupted around whether a low-fat or low-carbohydrate diet is better for weight loss. Going beyond this debate are questions around whether certain fatty acids are worse for promoting insulin resistance, inflammation, and obesity. The overall evidence suggests that lauric acid from coconut oil, and oleic acid from olive oil are less likely to promote insulin resistance, inflammation and fat storage, compared to the fats from butter and palm oil. Lauric acid and oleic acid are more likely to be burned for energy, and less likely to be stored as body fat. PUFAs such as linoleic acid found in vegetable oils, may contribute to obesity, whereas omega-3 PUFAs may be protective. Both olive oil as part of a Mediterranean diet, and omega-3 from fish and fish oil have been proven to reduce the risk of cardiovascular events.
www.ncbi.nlm.nih.gov/pmc/articles/PMC6140086/

But the most worrying aspect of too much saturated fat is the cancer connection:

Akhila Dandamudi et al. Dietary Patterns and Breast Cancer Risk: A Systematic Review. Anticancer Research Jun 2018, 38 (6) 3209- 3222.

Seventeen case-control studies found that vegetables were consistently found to be protective against breast cancer whereas saturated fat and red and processed meats were consistently found in patterns associated with increased breast cancer risk.

https://ar.iiarjournals.org/content/38/6/3209.long

Bojková B, Winklewski PJ, Wszedybyl-Winklewska M. Dietary Fat and Cancer - Which Is Good, Which Is Bad, and the Body of Evidence. Int J Mol Sci. 2020;21(11):4114. Published 2020 Jun 9.

A meta-analysis of case-control studies showed that olive oil consumption was associated with lower odds of having any type of cancer. In a prospective cohort study with 16 years of follow- up (521,120 individuals), replacement of just 5% of the saturated fatty acids with plant MUFAs resulted in an 11% decrease in cancer mortality. Nuts as another source of MUFAs may decrease cancer risk. Substantial evidence supports the widespread opinion that extra virgin olive oil should be the fat of choice when it comes to human health.

www.ncbi.nlm.nih.gov/pmc/articles/PMC7312362/

20.
MAN BOOBS

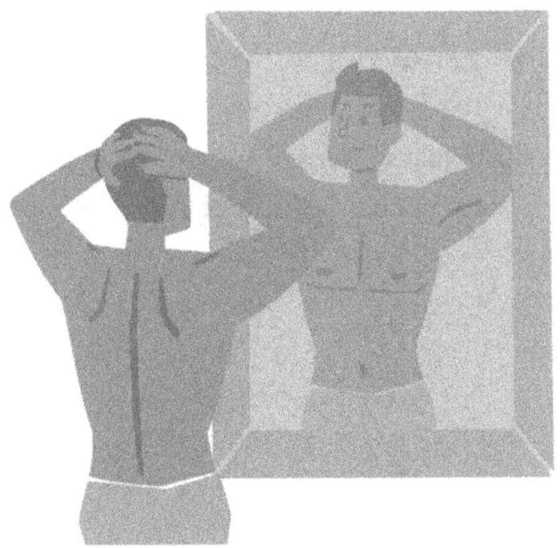

Man boobs are all about oestrogen. Yes, men can have oestrogen too! But naturally produced oestrogen in men should be broken down, so it does not encourage the growth of breast tissue. When oestrogen is not broken down it can encourage the growth of visceral fat and the development of 'man boobs'.

One of the factors that encourages man boobs is alcohol, which interferes with the liver's ability to break down oestrogen. A zinc deficiency can be a problem too, as it encourages testosterone to turn into oestrogen. Being overweight has a similar effect.

Oestrogen levels can also rise due to the presence of certain environmental pollutants linked to plastic. These are known as "xeno-oestrogens"; they include PCBs, BPA, BPS, BHA, dioxin and phthalates, and are thousands of times more potent than natural oestrogen. Plastics are extensively used for food packaging, bottled drinks, tetrapacks and to line the inside of food cans.

Water supplies can be contaminated with xeno-oestrogens, and eating fish that has been exposed to these hormone- disrupting pollutants can also be a source of contamination.

To prevent man boobs it is advisable to avoid consuming food or drink that has been stored or heated in plastic. 'Boil in the bag', and microwave ready meals are not recommended. Xeno-oestrogens can leach more rapidly into bottled water if plastic water bottles are left out in the sun. Bottled water has also been shown to contain high levels of plastic micro-particles.

21.
CONCLUSIONS: WHAT DOES THE RESEARCH REALLY SAY?

Yes, you'll find research studies stating that replacing all your carb calories with saturated fat, fish and meat doesn't appear to do you any harm, and will help you lose weight. The existence of these studies isn't disputed.

But if you look at the meta-analyses - the review studies which meticulously look at ALL the dieting research, and compare the use of these newer regimes with normal low-calorie diets, they don't come out any better. And the researchers all agree that they don't know what the long-term health effects of the extreme low-carb variants might be. They always conclude that more research is needed.

Even if a diet is only intended for short-term use to achieve a target weight, it is well known that the most difficult part of dieting is keeping the weight off once you have lost it. Constantly returning to an unbalanced form of dieting is likely to unbalance your health, and hasten the onset of age-related diseases.

What is most worrying about the trend towards carbo-phobia is the replacement of healthy carbs with meat and saturated fat. Both are relatively poor sources of nutrients, and meat is a kidney stressor. Displacing healthy carbs like those in legumes, carrots, fruit and whole-grains, with foods that contribute none of the antioxidants and phytonutrients that help to protect us from disease, is an experiment that you may come to regret.

So, what's the solution?

Yes, if your body no longer responds to simply restricting calories, it's likely you are becoming insensitive to insulin, producing too much of it, and it is blocking your ability to burn body fat. To control insulin you would benefit from avoiding sugars and starches (white flour and other refined grains) completely. Removing every single trace of other carbohydrates from your diet won't work any better for you, and means avoiding health-giving foods.

As stated by a growing number of experts, the most effective weight loss diet is the whole-food plant-based diet. If you use this as your main eating plan, plus calorie restriction, (eg. soup-based meals) and include an intermittent fasting schedule to aid fat burning, your weight loss plan will be sustainable, health-giving, and effective. You will avoid the carbs that have the worst insulin-stimulating effect, and by replacing most of your main meals with soup, you will be much less likely to fall by the wayside due to hunger.

Soup dieting is wonderful for helping you keep the calorie count low without constantly feeling hungry. Adding beans or lentils to those soups will also load you up with fantastic soluble fibre, the kind that controls appetite and helps to prevent insulin spikes.

Oats also provide soluble fibre. They fill you up quickly so you don't need to eat much, they're a good source of protein, and they're a far better source of vitamins and minerals than meat.

You can also achieve ketosis with a whole-food plant-based diet. just spend a few days from time to time eating nothing but leafy green soup, avocados, nuts, and olive or coconut oil, or use a fasting schedule like the 16:8 or 5:2 methods described earlier.

Don't forget to boost your calorie intake to normal levels once a week to keep up your metabolism, and exercise vigorously the day after, while your metabolism is still high. This really does make a difference.

The meal suggestions which I provide in the next sections give easy ways to get started on a whole-food plant-based, soup-rich diet, and act as a template which you can adapt and re-use. You will also find meal suggestions, recipes and links to useful food preparation sites and videos on my website www.modern-naturopathy.com.

What about fish and dairy products?

Some types of so-called "oily fish" are a good source of vitamin D, and the oils are the healthy omega-3 variety. But so are the oils from walnuts. On the other hand, walnuts don't raise the acid levels in your body like meat and fish do.

If you are fond of fish, a small serving once a week will not undo the benefits of your whole-food plant-based diet.

Dairy products can also provide a little vitamin D, and they are not as acid-forming as meat and fish. But for an awful lot of people they are a trigger of inflammatory problems, from migraine, to arthritis, asthma or even chronic constipation. It is well worth seeing how you feel if you avoid dairy products completely for a few months, and then only eat them occasionally.

We really don't need to get our calcium from dairy products. Much of the world's oriental population eats no dairy products at all because they are genetically not able to digest them after babyhood.

22.
TIME-SAVING TIPS

Soup is the way to go if you want to lose weight quickly without feeling hungry all the time. Soup doesn't have to be a smooth puree - it's much better with plenty of chunks.

Beans and lentils make a wonderful soup base. They are low in calories, high in soluble fibre, filling, satisfying, a good source of protein, and rich in iron, zinc and other vitamins and minerals. Buying beans in cans can work out expensive. and some brands contain sugar. It's better to buy dried beans. They need to be soaked overnight in water mixed with a teaspoon of baking soda before cooking. But if you cook a whole packet you can freeze what you don't need.

I cook beans in a pressure cooker, which takes less than ten minutes. If you don't have one, you'll have to allow an hour or two.

How to cook dried beans

Cover with at least four times their volume in water, stir in a teaspoon of baking soda (bicarbonate of soda) and leave overnight. Next day, throw away the soaking water, place the beans, well covered with fresh water, in a pressure cooker, bring to full steam, and leave on a low to medium heat for about 6 minutes. Remove the pressure cooker from the heat and leave until it has cooled down enough for you to open the lid. Try eating a bean to ensure that it is tender. If not, return the beans to the pan and cook for a little longer. You may need to experiment a few times to get the right degree of bean tenderness.

Pressure-cooking breaks down the poisonous lectins found in raw beans. If you do not have a pressure cooker, boil them fast for at least 10 minutes after soaking and before simmering or slow-cooking.

To freeze, allow the beans to cool, drain them, then spread them out on a baking tray. Once frozen, bang the tray to loosen the beans, then transfer them to freezer bags.

Cooking lentils

Lentils are so easy to cook, and make substantial, nutritious, low-calorie one-pot meals with very little effort. Use half a cup of uncooked lentils per serving. Put the lentils in a large pan and add about four times their volume of boiling water plus a little olive oil to stop them frothing up too much. Never add salt at this stage, as it will toughen them. Bring to the boil and cover the pan loosely (I put a spoon between the pan and the lid to help stop them boiling over). Simmer gently for 25-40 minutes, depending on the type of lentils, stirring occasionally. Red lentils take only 25 minutes. Brown, green or yellow lentils take 30 to 40 minutes. My favourites are the flat green ones.

Lentils boil over easily, so it's a good idea to use a pan several sizes larger than you would normally need.

To freeze cooked lentils, allow them to cool and put portions in freezer-proof containers.

23.
BREAKFAST

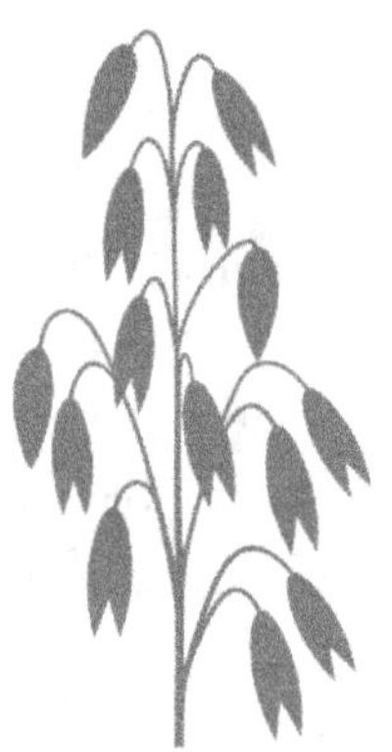

Oats are the ideal breakfast, so quick and nutritious. I promise they will not make you fat or unbalance your blood sugar. Yes, they are a source of carbohydrate, but it's superfood carbohydrate bound up with dietary fibre of the best possible type, and loaded with vitamins and minerals that support your metabolism. Oats are

- A good source of protein
- High in soluble fibre to help lower cholesterol, balance blood sugar, suppress appetite and help you stay full on less calories

- Rich in B vitamins, magnesium and other minerals
- A good source of the eye-protection nutrients lutein and zeaxanthin
- Oats contain powerful natural anti-inflammatory compounds called aventhramides.

Quick oatmeal bowl

Use 1/3rd cup of fine oatmeal per serving, mixed with 1/2 cup of water. Stir in a small handful of raisins and a small handful of pistachio kernels or crushed walnuts. You don't need to add any milk, since the oats make their own milk. You can buy fine oatmeal, but it's expensive. I prefer to grind rolled oats in a food processor.

Quick porridge

Use 1/3rd cup of rolled oats per serving, mixed with 1 cup water. Heat in a saucepan, stirring until thickened. Stir in some unsweetened plant milk of your choice, made from nuts, coconut, soy or even oats, then add raisins and chopped walnuts to taste. If you're trying to stay in ketosis after an overnight fast, an avocado smoothie is a good option. Blend an avocado with plant milk and a handful of walnuts.

Drinks

To keep your blood sugar in balance, anything you can do to encourage insulin sensitivity is helpful. Green tea has been shown to improve insulin sensitivity, and cinnamon can be added for an even better effect. Even just half a teaspoon of cinnamon per day has an anti- diabetic action. It is better not to add sweetener to drinks. Even relatively harmless alternative sweeteners like stevia can condition you to maintain a sugar craving. It doesn't take long to get used to drinks without sweetness.

24.
LIGHT MEALS AND LUNCHES

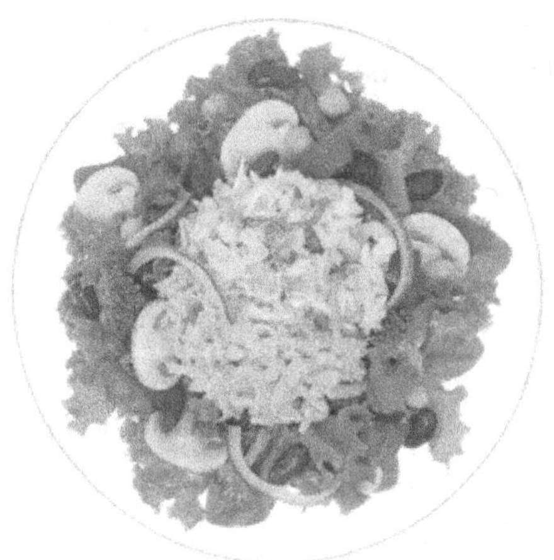

Oat wraps

Oat wraps are so simple to make, strong but soft. Spread with peanut butter and peach chunks and roll up for breakfast, or fill with hummus or mashed avocado and vegetable slaw for lunch.

For each wrap you will need:

- 1/3rd cup rolled oats and 1/3rd cup water

Preheat a large fry-pan with a heavy bottom, over a high heat. Whizz the two ingredients together in a blender until smooth, and immediately pour into the screaming hot pan. Quickly shake the pan to distribute the contents. You want to get a thin pancake like a crepe.

Turn the heat down to medium-hot and leave until the top has started to set and the bottom is strong enough for you to easily turn the pancake over with a spatula. Once turned over, cook for a minute or two until the bottom has little brown spots. Remove from the pan and if not consumed straight away, place the pancake between two kitchen dish towels to keep soft while you make some more.

Pumpernickel

I'm also going to recommend another healthy grain food for light meals and snacks: pumpernickel. This is a strong-tasting black rye bread that's loaded with vitamins, minerals and phytonutrients. Due to its strong taste, pumpernickel is best used to make open sandwiches topped with bean pâté and shredded salad vegetables. You can also eat it with a cup of instant soup made with miso paste, or a bean and vegetable salad with vinaigrette dressing or mayonnaise.

Miso paste is a healthy, vitamin-rich savoury Japanese paste used for flavouring soup, or you can just add it to a cup of boiling water. It is available in most supermarkets.

Instead of dairy butter, I would recommend an omega-3 rich vegan butter such as Earth Balance in the USA, or Naturli in Europe. These taste amazingly like real butter and can be used in just the same way.

To make bean pâté, cook some beans as previously described, or, if using canned beans, heat them in their liquid to soften them, then drain. While still warm, place in a food processor with some coconut oil, seasoning and any herbs or spices you like. Whizz until smooth. I use white cannellini beans or butterbeans (aka lima beans). The coconut oil is there to firm up the bean pâté once it has cooled in the fridge.

Avocados also make a delicious snack. I like them with a little olive oil and garlic vinaigrette.

25.
MAIN MEALS

In this section I'd like to concentrate on soup and soupy meals; warm liquid mixed with food, especially with the soluble fibre found in legumes and vegetables, helps to slow down your digestion and keep you feeling full.

These are the methods I use all the time to make my own soups. Hopefully once you've got the basic technique you'll be able to make soup with any veggies you have in your fridge, without needing to consult a recipe book.

Notes:

1. I prefer to use beans I have cooked myself, as I like them quite soft, almost on the point of breaking apart.

2. Just eyeball the vegetable quantity. How much do you think you can eat?

3. Since these are intended to be one-pot meals, the portions are meant to be larger than a normal soup serving.

Ingredients for 2-3 portions of soup

You will need:

2 cups of cooked beans or lentils

1 medium onion, chopped

1/4 cup olive oil

Flavourings to taste: e.g. garlic, herbs, lemon juice, chilli, tomato paste

Bouillon powder or a stock cube

Vegetables of your choice, shredded or roughly chopped. Cabbage or kale, leeks, parsley and carrots work well. Use a frozen veg mix if you're in a hurry.

Method

Using a large saucepan or a wok, gently soften the chopped onion in the olive oil for a few minutes over a low heat, keeping a lid on the pan. Add the shredded vegetables, stir and replace the lid. We are aiming to soften and collapse them. Keep an eye on the vegetables. Keep stirring, and add a dash of water if the pan gets dry.

Meanwhile, make the soup base. If using beans, liquidize one cup of cooked beans (eg. borlotti or cannellini beans) with 3 cups of hot vegetable bouillon or stock. I like to use a stick (hand-held) blender for this. Reserve the other cup of beans.

If using lentils, liquidize all the lentils into the 3 cups of stock/bouillon.

When the vegetables have collapsed and started to soften, pour the blended bean or lentil liquid into the pan and add any other chosen flavourings like dried herbs. If using beans, also add the reserved cup of unblended cooked beans. Check the consistency; ideally there should be just enough liquid in the pan to almost cover the vegetables. If there isn't enough liquid, top up with boiling water.

Bring the pan to the boil and simmer very gently until the vegetables are tender. Taste and correct the seasoning before serving. If you want to brighten the flavour, add a little lemon juice.

You can make endless permutations with this recipe. Variations include adding chopped fresh tomatoes just before serving, using oriental flavours like ginger and coriander leaf (cilantro), mirin and tamari, and unusual vegetable combinations like mooli (daikon) radish and broccoli.

Don't be mean with the parsley. An enormous bunch chops up quite small and when cooked adds enormous flavour and nutrition. Parsley is very good for your kidneys.

Pea pasta

If you haven't come across pea pasta, you may find this a very welcome addition to your weight loss regime. It is now available in the "Free From" section of most supermarkets, and is basically pasta made from pea protein. It's an excellent low-carb alternative to normal pasta. Cook according to the directions on the packet, and add a tomato-based pasta sauce like you normally would. Pea pasta is very filling. I find I only need to eat half as much as usual. You could also add it to soup, but I would advise to cook it separately first.

What about potatoes?

As you know, potatoes are a starchy vegetable, so are frowned on by authors of low-carb diets. It's true that potatoes can add a lot of carbohydrate to a meal, but only if you serve them as a main component.

A small potato diced up with other vegetables is not harmful, and adds several grams of protein.

One of my favourite meals is half a cauliflower cut small, plus a thinly-sliced potato and a tablespoon of olive oil, simmered with a cup of water until the liquid has almost all evaporated. Stir in some nutmeg and oat cream - delicious!

Desserts

Oranges, cherries, plums, peaches, apricots, melon, strawberries, raspberries and blackberries are the lowest carb fruits. Don't skimp on nutritious foods like fruit - they provide antioxidants and phytonutrients that help to keep us disease-free.

Instead of dairy cream, try whizzing some unsalted, rinsed raw cashew nuts with a can of coconut milk. Add a little vanilla extract for added flavour. Leave for a few minutes and it will start to thicken. This is a truly delicious combination!

For a refreshing soft drink to accompany your meal, mix fresh fruit juice 50:50 with sparkling water.

Note from the Author

I'd love to know how you get on!
Drop me a line in the chat forum at my website
www.modern-naturopathy.com.
You'll also find lots of information there on
whole-food plant-based dieting. Plus,
Use the Research link to find out what's new,
Look for the pages with links to recipe sites,
easy recipes and recipe videos,
Use the Ask A Naturopath forum to post your questions
and I will personally answer when I can.

Wishing you success with your dieting

Linda

Linda Lazarides BA(Hons)
Principal and Founder
School of Modern Naturopathy
BCM Waterfall
London WC1N 3XX
United Kingdom

www.modern-naturopathy.com
Internet-based training courses

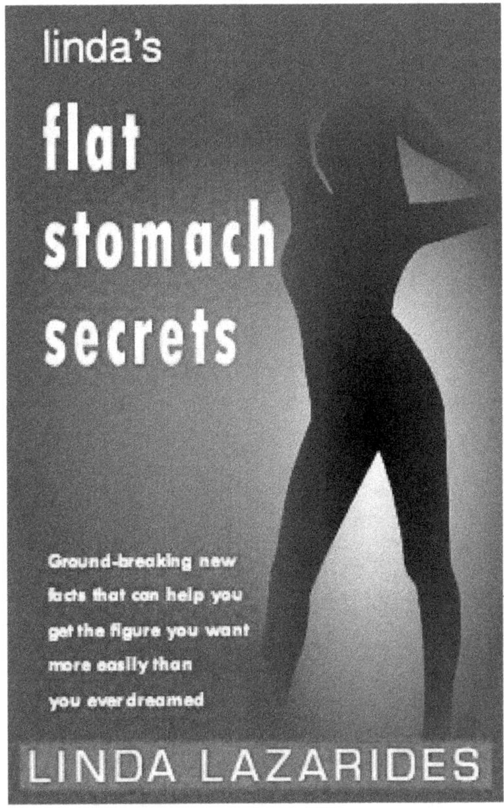

Linda Lazarides is a holistic practitioner - she likes to look at the big picture. So she went on a quest to discover all the reasons why a tummy bulge can be so hard to lose. Once you know why a problem occurs you can start to look for the solution. Altogether she found FIVE different causes. She also found what she believes are the very best methods to deal with each of these five causes. If you follow the five-pronged approach in this book, you will massively improve your prospects of getting a flat stomach.

On the next page is an extract from Chapter 2 of *Linda's Flat Stomach Secrets*.

CHAPTER 2

INTERNAL FAT
THE ALIEN WITHIN

We all know about the fat on the outside of your stomach that you can pinch between finger and thumb. Some of us can pinch more than others! Have you ever wondered why the size of your waist doesn't seem to match the amount of fat you can pinch? I used to know a woman named Maggie who was overweight probably by about 30 lbs. One day I saw her in a bikini and was completely amazed that her stomach was absolutely flat, even though it had a bit of fat on it. Only recently have I discovered how that is possible. There are actually two kinds of tummy fat. One is external (the fat you can see and hold on to). The other is internal. Internal fat is also known as "visceral fat". It accumulates inside the abdomen, between the internal organs, and makes the belly protrude or stick out at the front. Maggie's stomach was flat because she had very little "internal fat".

A tummy with a lot of internal fat is also known as a "pot-belly" or sometimes a "beer belly". If you have this problem, you can measure how severe it is by calculating your "waist to hip ratio". The higher the ratio, the more internal fat you have.

Calculate your waist-to-hip ratio (WHR)

You will need a measuring tape and a calculator

1. Gently breathe out and relax.
2. Without holding in your tummy, measure your waist circumference.

(Your waist is at the halfway point between the base of your ribs and your hip-bone.) You can use inches or centimeters. Do not pull the tape too tight.

3. Measure your hip circumference around the fullest part of your bottom (butt).

4. Using your calculator, divide the waist measurement by the hip measurement.

For example, if your waist is 36 inches and your hips are 42 inches, then divide 36 by 42. The answer is 0.85, which is your waist-to-hip ratio.

People with a high WHR are considered to be at risk of getting a heart attack, stroke or diabetes. The WHR is thought to predict a person's risk of these problems more accurately than the overall body weight or even the body mass index (BMI). Further alarming research shows that fat accelerates ageing, probably by speeding up the unravelling of basic genetic structures inside cells. Writing in the medical journal *The Lancet* in 2005, Professor Tim Spector and his team at St Thomas' Hospital, London, and the University of Medicine and Dentistry of New Jersey, studied more than 1,000 women, and found that the more people weigh, the older their cells appear. Obesity adds the equivalent of almost nine years of age to a person's body, and smoking has similar harmful effects. Use the chart below to assess your WHR.

Waist-to-Hip Ratio Chart

	Men	Women
Low	0.95 or less	0.80 or less
Medium	0.96 to 1.0	0.81 to 0.85
High (high risk of heart attack, stroke or diabetes)	1.0 or higher	0.85 or higher

How your "internal alien" makes you crave food

It's bad enough that internal fat expands your waistline. But this type of fat also has some nasty characteristics that make it very undesirable.

1. Internal fat is like an alien from outer space, protecting its own growth and development by giving you addictive food cravings. It does this by deactivating a substance called leptin which your body produces to suppress your appetite when you've had enough to eat. (NB: Fructose can also deactivate leptin.)

2. Internal fat also protects itself from destruction. When it reaches a certain level it makes your body produce more insulin. The presence of Insulin protects this fat from being broken down and used for fuel.

3. The more internal fat you have, the closer you are to developing high blood pressure and diabetes. Nothing predicts these diseases better than your waist size. If your waist circumference is more than 40 inches (100 cm) then you so close to developing these problems that you may already have them.

The "alien" analogy is not so far off. Scientists are indeed saying that internal fat can take on a life of its own. Unlike the fat under your skin, internal abdominal fat is highly active, a living, throbbing organ that produces particles which attack good health. These particles are known as cytokines. They cause inflammation and swelling and are blamed for a wide range of health problems from heart disease to diabetes, dementia (senility) and rheumatoid arthritis. In fact, internal fat is so strongly linked with diabetes, that in animal experiments carried out at the Albert Einstein College of Medicine, New York, in 2002, the pre-diabetic condition known as "metabolic syndrome" was reversed when internal fat was surgically removed from the animals' abdomens.

Internal fat starts to affect men in middle age when their testosterone levels go down and their oestrogen levels go up. The term "beer gut" is very accurate, since alcohol decreases the ability of the liver to break down oestrogen. If a man's liver cannot break down oestrogen he will have more of it in his system. This encourages both internal fat and the development of "man boobs". Men with a zinc deficiency may also be prone to developing these problems, as zinc deficiency encourages the conversion of testosterone to oestrogen. Overall body weight plays a part too. Testosterone in overweight men gets converted to oestrogen more rapidly.

In women, on the other hand, oestrogen seems to offer some protection against the development of internal fat, as this type of fat mostly develops after the menopause, when oestrogen levels decline and the proportion of male hormones rises. Before the menopause, women store fat in their hips and thighs, but after the menopause, fat migrates to their belly.

What Causes Internal Fat?

So far we know of two main causes. The first is a hormone produced by your adrenal glands (situated above your kidneys). Its name is cortisol and it helps your body to cope with stress.

Stress

Researchers have known for some time that people with Cushing's syndrome - a disease in which levels of cortisol are very high - seem to have very large waistlines due to large amounts of internal fat. In healthy people, cortisol levels rise when you are under stress. Although all of us are exposed to stress, some people produce more cortisol than others when they are under stress. Also, some people become stressed more easily than others, or fail to learn to adapt to stressful situations. So in 2000, Dr Elissa Epel and her colleagues at Yale University decided to investigate whether people who get stressed very easily, have larger waistlines.

Dr Epel measured the WHR of 59 white women and, over a period of several days, gave them laboratory stress tests and then tested the amounts of cortisol they produced when they were under stress. About half the women had a high WHR and the other half had a low WHR. The results were astounding. Women with a big waistline did indeed seem to get stressed more easily and produced more cortisol than women with a small waistline.

The researchers concluded that women who are more nervous, or more vulnerable to stress, are more likely to find that their waistline expands as they get older. This happens even if they don't consume any more calories, and even if the rest of their body is not particularly fat. Of course, genetics, other hormones and lifestyle can also play a role. Smoking, alcohol and lack of exercise tend to increase internal fat, say the researchers, whereas getting sufficient sleep and exercise can actually reduce it. Their findings were reported in the journal Psychosomatic Medicine in 2000. Sleep also helps to slow down the ageing process. People who don't sleep enough have higher levels of the cytokines which we now know to be the promoters of diabetes and heart disease.

Sugar

Many of us turn to sugary foods when we are under stress even though we all know that sugar is a very concentrated source of calories and liable to make us put on weight. Any sugar which your body cannot use gets turned into fat quite quickly. Most of the sugar we consume is hidden in sugary foods and soft drinks or sodas. It's very easy to put on a lot of extra weight if you indulge in these foods and don't take enough exercise to burn off the extra calories.

When you consume sugar, it's not just the calories that make you put on weight. A much more serious fattening effect comes from the hormonal and metabolic changes that take place when you consume sugar. Consuming sugary foods and drinks makes you produce a hormone called insulin, and the more sugary the items you consume, the more insulin you produce. Consuming foods which are high in both fat and sugar, such as chocolate and ice cream, makes you produce even more insulin. Insulin makes you put on weight because it increases the amount of fat that goes into storage and stops you from breaking down fat to use as energy.

As we know, fat can go into storage under your skin, or inside your abdomen, where it is known as internal fat. The amount of internal fat you store depends depends on the type of sugar you consume, so at this point we need to learn a little bit about sugar. The sugar crystals that you buy in packets or which are added to food usually consist of a chemical known as sucrose. Sucrose itself consists of two individual sugars bound together, whose names are fructose and glucose. When you eat sucrose, you are eating 50 per cent glucose and 50 per cent fructose - half and half. Your digestion breaks the sucrose down into these two individual sugars which then enter your bloodstream.

Glucose travels around your body and can be used as fuel or turned into fat. But fructose does not travel around. It stays in your abdomen, and your liver turns it into internal abdominal fat. This discovery is quite recent. In 2009 doctors Stanhope and Havel at the University of California carried out research in which they asked two groups of people to drink beverages every day in addition to their normal diet. The first group had to drink beverages sweetened with glucose and the other group had to drink beverages sweetened with fructose. After ten weeks, both groups had gained the same amount of weight. But while the glucose group gained fat evenly throughout their body, the fructose group were found to have gained substantially more internal fat.

Does sugar really give you energy?

Many people believe the old saying that sugar "gives you energy". But US bodybuilding and fitness guru John Parrillo explains how fructose actually robs you of energy. It does this by forcing your body to turn many foods into fat instead of turning them into glycogen - precious fuel for your muscles. When muscles lack glycogen, you feel heavy and lethargic. When your muscles have plenty of glycogen, you feel energetic and full of stamina.

Parrillo has carried out many nutritional experiments with bodybuilders. When a bodybuilder gets close to a contest, his (or her) body fat levels get so low that any tiny change becomes immediately apparent and is easy to measure. This state is ideal for experiments, so Parrillo has been able to measure the effects of many different foods. In one of his early tests he removed 300-calories-worth of rice from the bodybuilders' daily diet and replaced it with 300-calories-worth of bananas. To his amazement they started to gain fat. He continued the experiment for two weeks and the athletes continued to gain fat. Then he stopped the bananas and put the rice back in. The fat started to reduce. These results were mind-blowing, as they thoroughly explode the myth that calories are calories and the type of calorie makes no difference to your body weight.

Parrillo knew that in order to work, muscles need glycogen, which is a form of carbohydrate that they can store and utilise as fuel. If you want to feel energetic and burn off the calories in your food rather than turn them into fat, you have to eat carbs that drip-feed glycogen into your muscles. Complex carbohydrates such as bread and rice (preferably whole-grain), pasta, potatoes, beans and oatmeal are very good at this, as they are broken down and absorbed slowly. On the other hand if you consume a soda or drink sweetened with corn syrup, or eat something sugary, the fructose in these items will hog the enzyme which other carbs need in order to become muscle glycogen. Fructose uses the enzyme to create lots of glycogen for the liver, but that glycogen can't be used by the muscles. So for the next few hours the muscles will get less glycogen, even if you have just done a workout and your muscles are weak and starved. The unused fructose becomes internal fat, and the carbs that should have become muscle glycogen are also made into fat. Result? More fat, less energy.

How To Reduce Internal Fat

Controlling Fructose

It you want to lose tummy fat and gain energy, it's clearly very important to avoid eating fructose-rich foods as much as possible. This means you have to check the labels of everything you consume. Most sweetened products such as ice cream, chocolate and desserts will have the word "sugar" listed in their ingredients. Sugar usually means sucrose, which as we know is half glucose and half fructose. It's not good, but there are sweeteners out there with even higher amounts of fructose. In recent years there has been a tendency to use corn syrup as a sweetener. It's very cheap, has a lot of sweetening power, and consists of 55 to 90 per cent fructose. Sometimes known as HFCS (high-fructose corn syrup) it is found in a wide variety of commercial, processed foods, especially soft drinks or sodas.

Fructose is often claimed to be a healthy option because it has a low glycaemic index - it doesn't raise blood sugar very much. But the reason for its low glycaemic index is that your liver quickly turns it into fat. Another so-called healthy option, agave nectar, is actually 56 to 92 per cent fructose, depending on the brand. Even honey is mostly fructose.

The Fructose Content of Common Sweeteners

Sweetener	Fructose grams/100g	Glucose grams/100g
Sucrose	50	50
Honey	40.9	35.7
Corn syrup	55 to 90	10 to 45
Agave nectar	56 to 92	8 to 44
Maple syrup	50	50

The table above shows a list of sweeteners and their glucose and fructose contents.

The following foods are likely to contain more fructose than glucose)
- Apple juice
- Pear juice (some tinned fruits are canned in pear juice)
- Items such as sodas and snack bars sweetened with corn syrup.

It's wise to avoid apple and pear juice because they are more concentrated sources of fructose than the actual fruits themselves. But there's no need to stop eating the fruits; a fresh apple or pear only contains a few grams of fructose, which is negligible.

All fruits contain fructose (another name for fructose is fruit sugar) but the following fruits are best as their fructose content is equal to or less than glucose:

* Stone fruit: apricot, nectarine, peach, plum

* Berry fruit: blueberry, blackberry, boysenberry, cranberry, raspberry, strawberry

* Citrus fruit: kumquat, grapefruit, lemon, lime, mandarin, orange, tangelo

* Other fruits: ripe banana, jackfruit, kiwi fruit, passion fruit, pineapple, rhubarb, tamarillo

Alternative sweeteners

If you intend to improve your waistline but are not ready to take up meditation or knitting instead of comfort food as an anti-stress therapy, you will have to find an alternative sweetener.

Artificial sweeteners

Artificial sweeteners may appear to be the answer, and perhaps they are ok if consumed in small amounts, very occasionally. Personally I would never eat or recommend these chemical products. I believe they cause stress to the liver, and can be difficult to metabolize. Some, such as aspartame - the chemical name for proprietary sweeteners used in hundreds of "low-calorie", "sugar-free" or "diet" products - have been linked with unpleasant health problems such as dizziness, recurring headaches and even seizures.

There's also new research to show that artificial sweeteners can increase cravings for sweets and other carbohydrates. Incredibly, researchers have found that using sweeteners can lead to faster weight gain than consuming sugary foods and drinks.

A 2008 Purdue University study published in the journal Behavioral Neuroscience, reported that rats fed with artificially-sweetened yoghurt gained more weight than rats given yoghurt containing natural sugar. The rats which were fed artificial sweeteners ended up eating more and adding extra body fat compared with the rats whose yoghurt was sweetened with glucose sugar.

But it's not just animals who suffer these effects. A major American research study was carried out in 1988 on 80,000 women aged 50 to 69 years. Those who used artificial sweeteners were compared with those who did not. Regardless of their initial weight, the women who used the sweeteners put on more weight per year than the women who did not use them. (Reported in Appetite journal, Vol 11, 1988.)

It seems that sweeteners may make you put on weight because they increase your appetite. Another study was carried out in 1990 at the Monell Chemical Senses Center, Philadelphia. For 15 minutes, 10 men and 10 women chewed chewing gum sweetened with four different doses of aspartame. Their subsequent hunger was then compared with groups given either nothing or unsweetened chewing gum. The gum containing the least aspartame did not significantly increase appetite, but the gum containing moderate concentrations did. The gum containing the highest concentration of aspartame initially reduced appetite but this was followed by a sustained increase in hunger ratings. (Reported in the Physiology and Behavior journal, volume 47, 1990.)

Researchers have been trying to explain why this hunger occurs. It seems that your gut has "taste" cells which taste sugar and artificial sweeteners through the same mechanisms used by the taste cells of the tongue. The gut taste cells regulate secretion of insulin and hormones that regulate appetite. Whether you eat sugar, or whether you just eat something that tastes like sugar, your body will produce similar amounts of insulin. The insulin searches for the expected sugar, but when it is not found it eliminates some of your blood sugar instead. As your blood sugar drops, you develop hunger cravings which subsequently make you eat more. (Artificial Sweeteners: Fat or Fiction? International Institute for Anti-Ageing, 2009.)

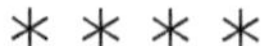

Packed with fascinating information, *Linda's Flat Stomach Secrets* explains the five causes of an expanding waistline and includes a comprehensive program and 7-day diet to begin to tackle it. You could lose as much as three inches from your waistline in three months. Discover

- How to avoid developing obsessive food cravings
- How to rebalance the hormones that control belly fat
- A cool way of walking that powerfully works out your tummy muscles at the same time
- What is intestinal plaque and how it can cause bloating
- A deep-cleansing routine to tackle bloating, gas and water retention.

Linda's Flat Stomach Secrets is available from good bookstores and online retailers.

THE SCHOOL OF MODERN NATUROPATHY

Have you ever thought about training as a naturopathic nutritionist? This is a natural health consultant who specializes in creating tailored health programs which can help individuals overcome common health problems and ailments.

Linda Lazarides teaches a one-year diploma course by distance learning, using a combination of specially written course modules and internet-based teaching. This course is accredited by major organizations in more than 20 countries. Upon successful completion, you would be qualified to work as a wellness counsellor, health coach, naturopathic nutritionist or nutrition advisor. You would be eligible to set up in private practice, or work in a health club, health food store or perhaps for a vitamin or natural products company.

If you plan to work as a writer or journalist, you would gain an in-depth understanding of holistic health which would greatly improve the quality of your books and articles and also make it much easier for you to find ideas and reliable information for articles to interest your readers.

Linda Lazarides is a master practitioner and founder of the British Association for Nutritional Therapy. In 1996 she helped the University of Westminster to set up the UK's first degree course in Nutritional Therapy. and previously for several years worked as a complementary practitioner for the British National Health Service. She has been a nutrition editor for the *International Journal of Alternative and Complementary Medicine*, an advisor to several national organizations, and has been invited to speak at parliamentary committees in the UK.

For more information about the
School of Modern Naturopathy
please visit
www.modern-naturopathy.com

www.ingramcontent.com/pod-product-compliance
Lightning Source LLC
Chambersburg PA
CBHW061725250726
48657CB00002B/768